ROB BATEZEL

My Life
with Mosaic Down Syndrome

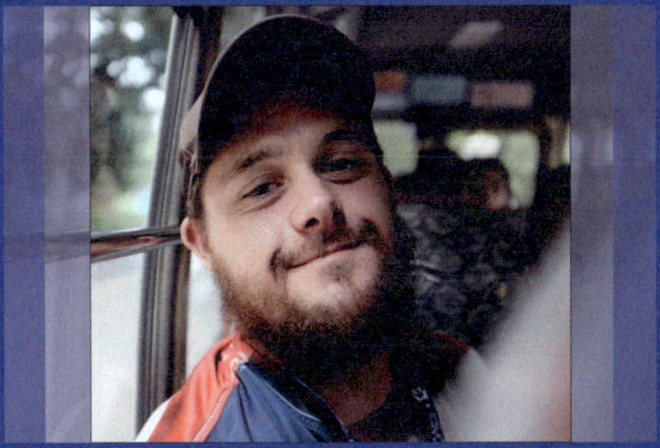

Rob in Hong Kong in 2016

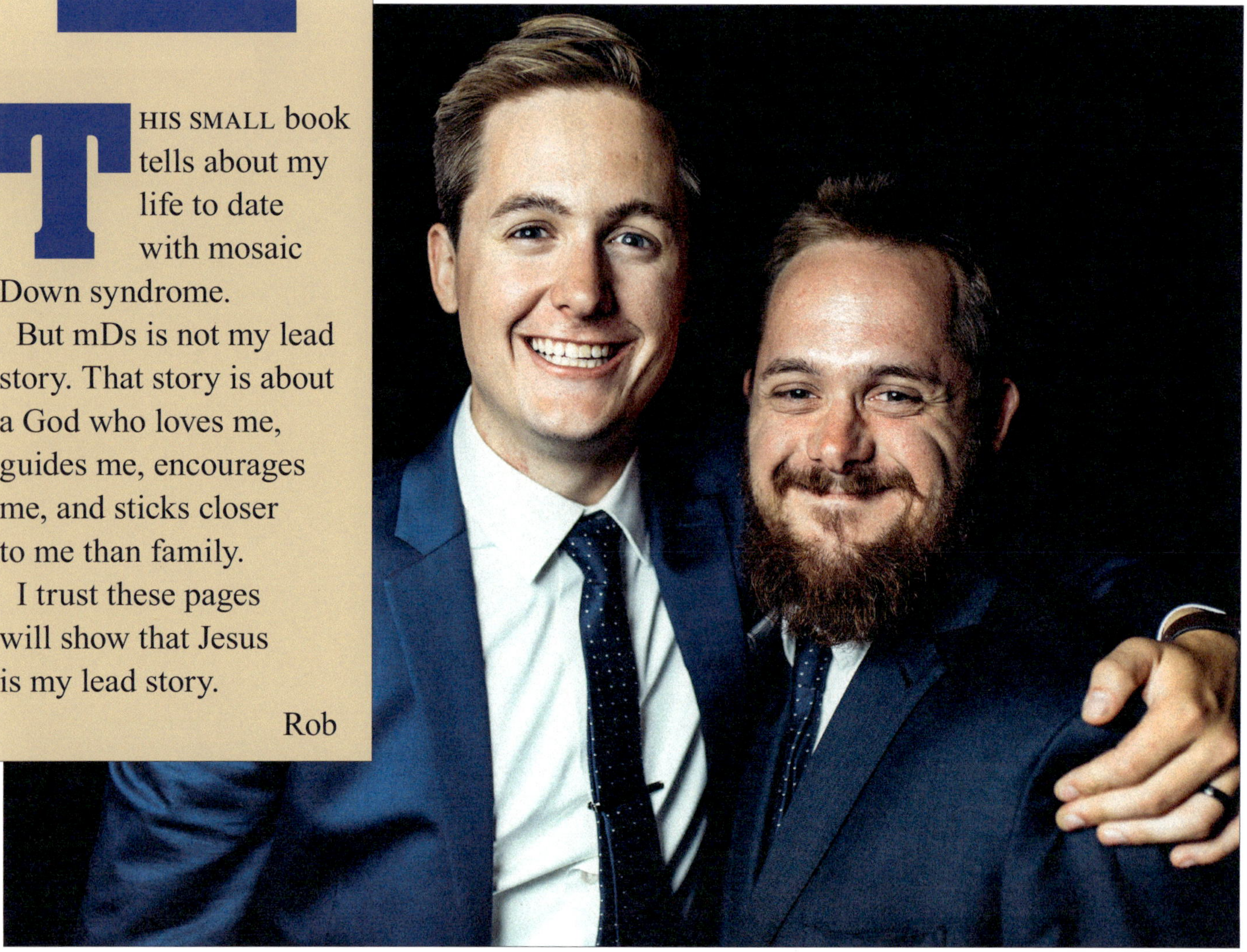

THIS SMALL book tells about my life to date with mosaic Down syndrome.

But mDs is not my lead story. That story is about a God who loves me, guides me, encourages me, and sticks closer to me than family.

I trust these pages will show that Jesus is my lead story.

Rob

Speaking of family...

Hold the asterisk. He's my brother.

by Casey Batezel

> *Therefore, since we are surrounded by such a great cloud of witnesses, let us throw off everything that hinders and the sin that so easily entangles. And let us run with perseverance the race marked out for us....*
>
> Hebrews 12:1 (NIV)

Casey (left) on his wedding day with his brother and best man, Rob.

THE WORLD can describe my brother Rob as a lot of things — high school graduate, welder, carpenter, reliable and competent teammate, jokester.

I can describe him as even more — encourager, generous soul, lover-of-submarines, child of God. Both are long lists — but neither mentions **mosaic Down syndrome** — mDs (where random cells have an extra chromosome). At least for me, that's intentional. Rob is more than a diagnosis.

I am a lot of things. I'm white, I'm a man, I'm right handed. But any success or failure I experience rises and falls on me — on Casey.

I've wanted the same for Rob. He's a lot of things, but his successes shouldn't be marked by an asterisk indicating "disabled due to mDs." His successes should be presented alone, in the context of Rob.

He regularly makes significant contributions to his world. He loves serving others, or getting to know somebody enough to give them a great gift. He knows everything about sports. He boldly presents his faith and unashamedly calls those around him to a greater life. These are the things that mark my brother.

I hope you will recognize small ways Rob's character can impact how you live. Not his character as defined by disability — but as Rob, a good man, my brother.

Our world doesn't need more division or labels. We need more good men and women who are willing to rise above and make a difference. Like Rob.

Early days

> *"I will be a Father to you, and you will be my sons and daughters, says the Lord Almighty."*
> 2 Corinthians 6:18 (NIV)

MY MOM went into premature labor on June 1, 1990 (the due date was July 22). The doctor admitted her to Wilford Hall USAF Medical Center in San Antonio and tried to stop the labor.

By June 5 my heart rate wasn't accelerating properly, and the doctor decided to deliver me. I arrived at 9:23 p.m. that day, measuring 5 1/2 pounds and 19 inches. My parents named me Robyn Davace (a blend of Horace and David, my paternal and maternal grandfathers).

I had blue eyes and brown hair. The pediatricians and neonatologist took me right away to the NICU (neonatal intensive care unit). During a physical exam, they noticed a simian crease on my right palm and decided to test me for Down syndrome.

They found that I had a rare form called **mosaic Down syndrome.** They said 40 percent of my cells had the extra 21st chromosome, according to buccal swab tests. Later blood tests lowered the ratio to 12 percent.

I was in the hospital for two and one-half weeks due to beta strep. I was on oxygen for one day. I also had jaundice and laryngeal/trachea malacia. At two months, I started physical and occupational therapy through CAMP (Children's Association for Maximum Potential) at Lackland AFB.

In July, I visited my ill grandfather in Hawaii. In October, I went to my first of many International Balloon Fiestas in Albuquerque, N.M.

In February 1991, Dad retired from the Air Force. I went to the ceremonies in my own little uniform tailored by a friend.

In April I got my first set of pressure-equalizing (PE) tubes. I eventually had eight sets, then stopped having ear infections when I went off milk at age 8.

In May, I mastered a commando belly-crawl and was on the move! Then I learned to crawl on all fours. Soon, I started cruising around furniture and learning to sit down from standing. I started walking at 16 months.

In August, we took a road trip of 6,000 miles. I loved seeing myself in a car mirror and playing with my Koosh Ball. We went to Albuquerque to see **Aunt Suzie** and her family. Later we visited friends in Washington, D.C., and Florida. I had a blast throughout the journey.

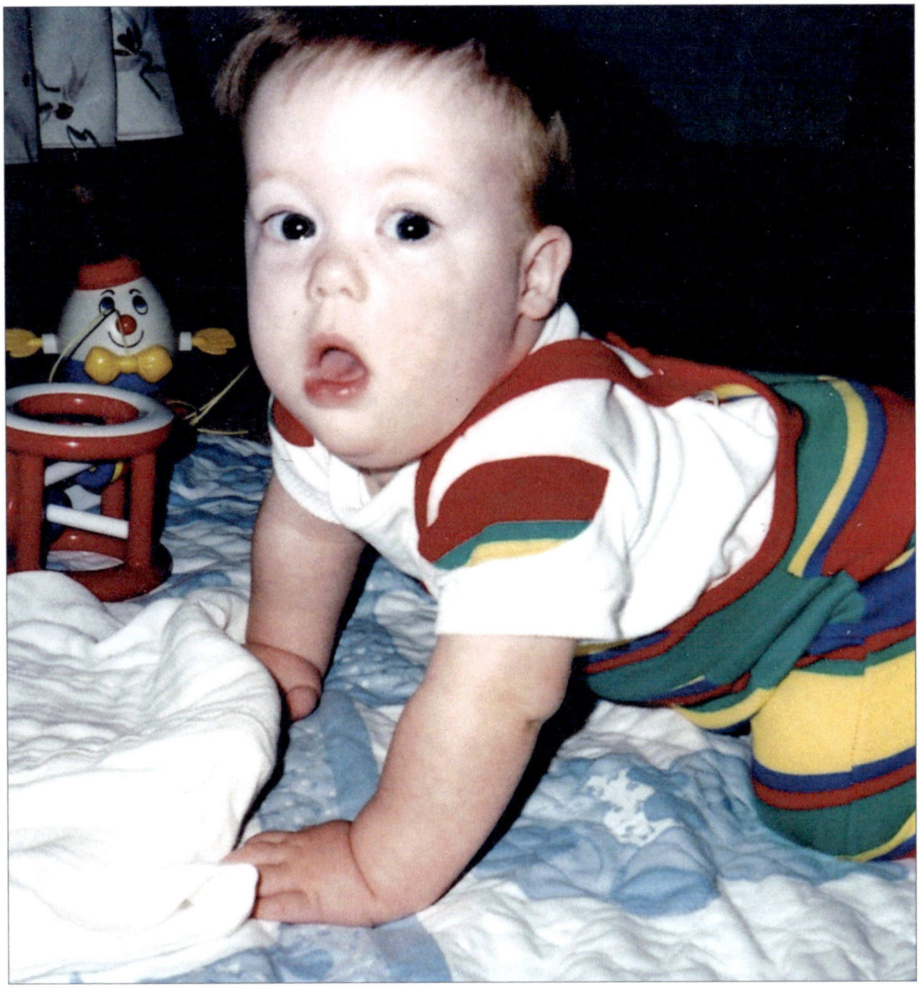

Rob ready to crawl at ten months.

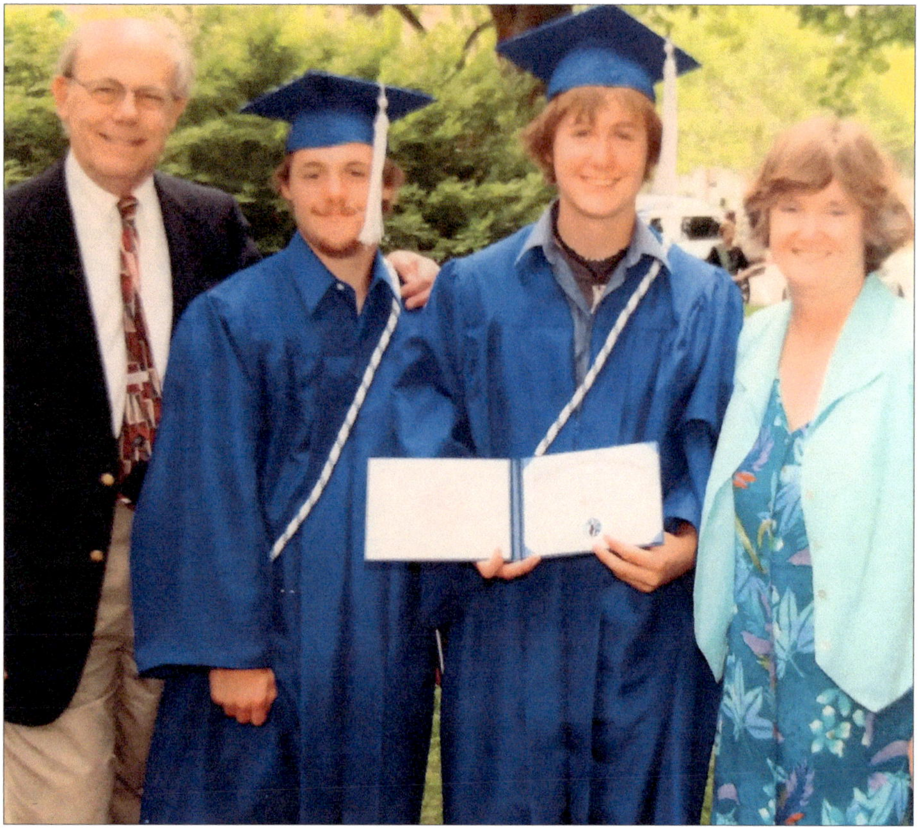

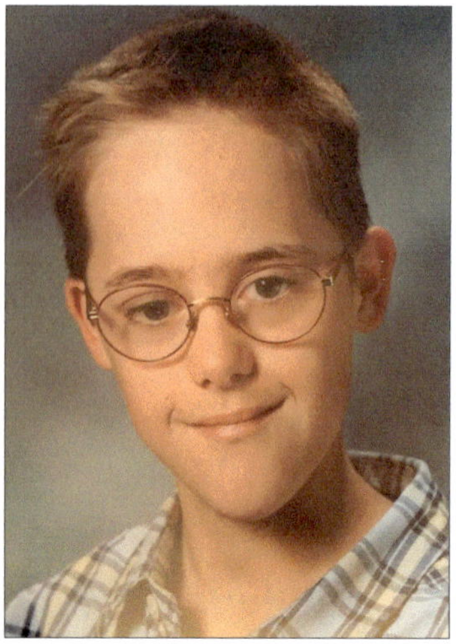

School days

Don't let your school struggles limit your career dreams.

Rob

Left: Rob and Casey at their May 2009 high school graduation. **Above:** Rob as a seventh-grader.

In San Antonio, I attended the city's pilot program for an inclusion preschool. The staff consisted of a special-education teacher, a speech/language pathologist and an occupational therapist.

On graduating preschool, I went to a full-day kindergarten at Braun Station Elementary School. It was a year-round program that was also the regional school for the deaf. Everyone learned to sign. I am a visual learner, so the program was perfect for me.

I was diagnosed as language- and learning-disabled, which warranted speech and language therapy and resource support. I also had apraxia. In third grade I was also diagnosed with attention deficit disorder without hyperactivity. I eventually tested out of being learning-disabled because my language scores had improved, but I was still able to get services authorized for my disability (Section 504 of the federal Rehabilitation Act of 1973).

In Fort Collins I attended fourth and fifth grades at Bauder Elementary School. I went on 14 field trips and built a model of Mesa Verde. I was in a social skills group and had speech and language therapy. I also got help with reading and math.

In sixth grade, I switched to PIONEER, an expeditionary learning school. My brother Casey skipped fifth grade to join me in the sixth grade at the new school.

At PIONEER we went on frequent field trips and multi-day camping trips to study nature and environmental issues. I loved the "hands-on" learning and the small class sizes (20:1). Two years before Casey and I graduated, PIONEER changed its name to Polaris Expeditionary Learning School.

While a junior, I joined a carpentry class for high school students through Front Range Community College (FRCC). The carpentry skills came in handy years later when I helped my brother and his wife remodel a house that was almost 100 years old.

As a senior, I joined a high school welding program at FRCC. I was chosen from among 25 students to learn tungsten inert gas (TIG) welding. I designed a model warship using computer-assisted design (CAD), then built it using my TIG welding skills. I christened it the USS Polaris (see centerfold) and presented it to the school as a class gift when Casey and I graduated in May 2009.

Scouts

> *Teach Scouts not how to get a living, but how to live.*
>
> Robert Baden-Powell

MY BROTHER Casey and I started in Cub Scouts as Tigers at Braun Station Elementary School in San Antonio. I went on to the rank of Bobcat in 1st grade, advancing to Wolf and Bear before our family moved to Colorado. I recall a trip with my pack to the Houston Space Center where we learned the history of the NASA space program. Back home, we built small cars and raced them at the annual Pinewood Derby in our school auditorium.

Casey and I continued in Cub Scouts after our move to Colorado. In due time I achieved Webelo rank. Both my parents were den leaders or assistant leaders.

I bridged to Boy Scout Troop 12 in 2002. I learned a huge amount from the amazing Scout leaders who helped me earn merit badges. I had to have 21 badges to reach Eagle Scout, the highest scouting rank.

As Scouts, we sold popcorn and hauled off neighbors' Christmas trees after the holiday season to raise money. I went to camps in Colorado, Wyoming and Nebraska. At one, I learned how to throw tomahawks and build a log cabin. Once we camped at the Air Force Academy in Colorado Springs and attended a cadet football game.

To become an Eagle, Scouts must complete a community service project. I decided to convert a long and wide drainage ditch at my school into an environmental wetlands (see centerfold). I raised the construction money by selling Interstate Batteries with the help of classmates. I also received a grant from the First National Bank in Fort Collins. One of my Scout leaders, a landscape architect named **Dana Leavitt,** helped me determine the plants and trees I would need. A generous gentleman in the community donated the hydroponics so that seed could be spread throughout the area. Local nurseries gave me a good deal on the plants and trees and donated tree straps and stakes. About 250 classmates and Scouts helped with the planting.

With great pride and satisfaction, I achieved the rank of Eagle Scout in June of 2006, just before turning 16.

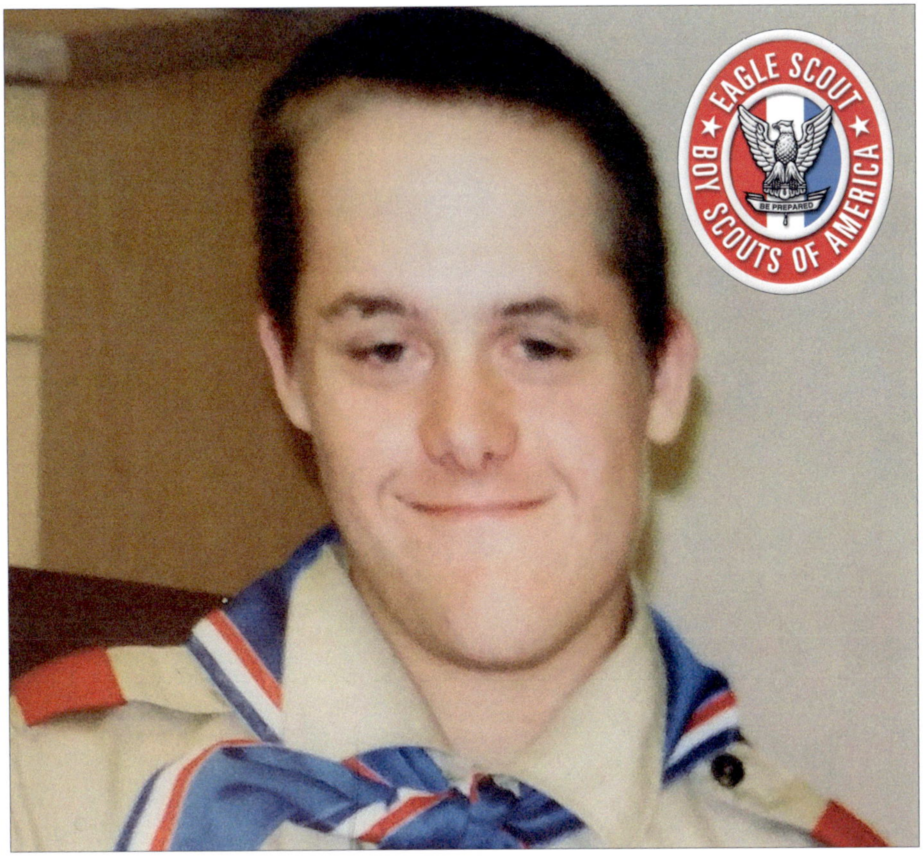

Eagle Scout Rob.

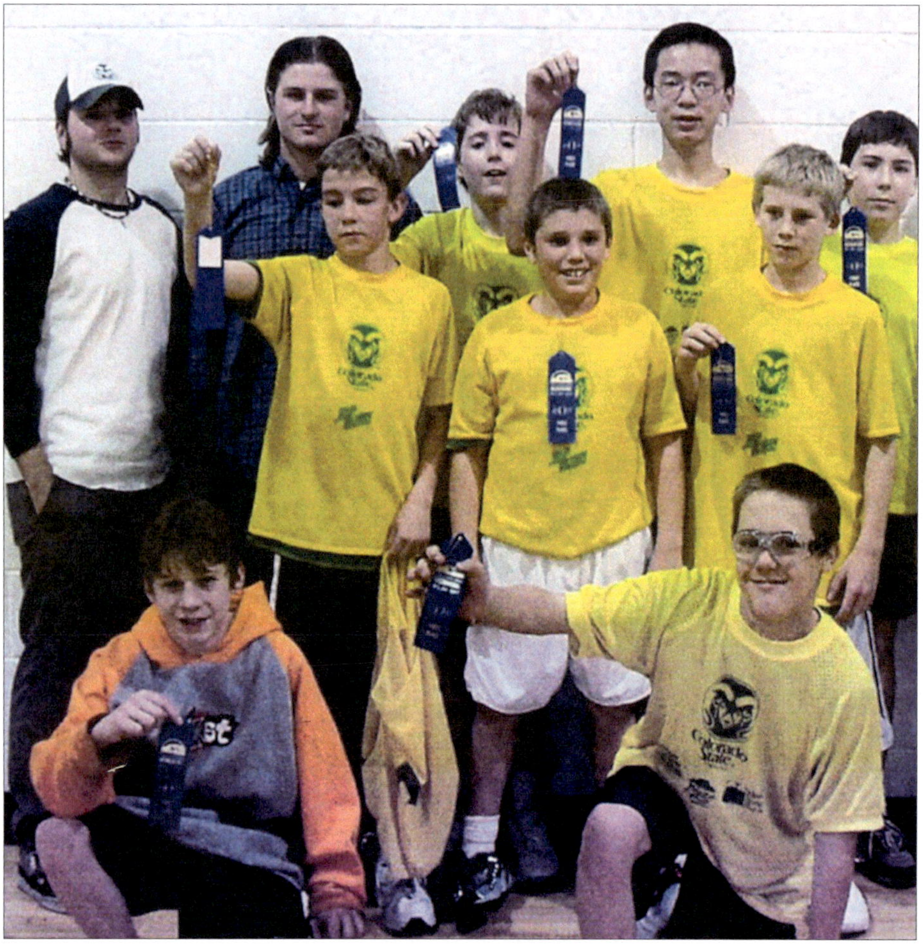

Sports/music

Sports and music often define the person you will become.

Rob

Left: *Rob and his basketball teammates in 7th grade in Fort Collins.* **Opposite:** *Rob at the drums in San Antonio.*

DURING THE years in San Antonio, I was able to do soccer, baseball and swimming. Because of our move to Fort Collins in June of 2000, I was unable to play any sports that summer since the team rosters were already filled.

I resumed basketball during my fourth-grade year. I learned the positions of small forward and power forward.

Starting in the sixth grade at PIONEER, I played basketball at nearby schools because PIONEER lacked its own teams. This began the era when I nailed the three-pointer. (In one game, a coach bragged that I made a three-pointer five feet beyond the three-point line!) I continued playing on city leagues during the rest of high school.

At Mesa State College in Grand Junction, Colo., I polished my basketball skills. On returning to college in Fort Collins, I started playing in church leagues. In one game, I made four three-pointers.

Music is as important to me as sports. I got my first keyboard when I was 2. I went on to play the recorder, guitar and drums.

At 6 and 7 respectively, my brother and I took piano lessons. The music teacher taught us to distinguish high from low notes as though they were "birds tweeting in the trees" and "lions rumbling in the jungle." Later, I experimented with the trombone and base guitar.

After moving to Colorado in 2000, we took private drum lessons both in our home and at a studio.

As an adult I continue to practice my bass at home and with a church group called Mill City Anchor.

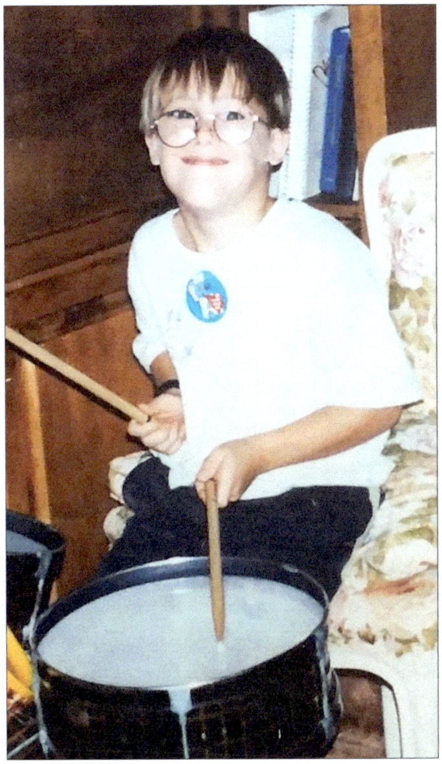

Rob practicing the drums in San Antonio.

THE WETLANDS AT PIONEER

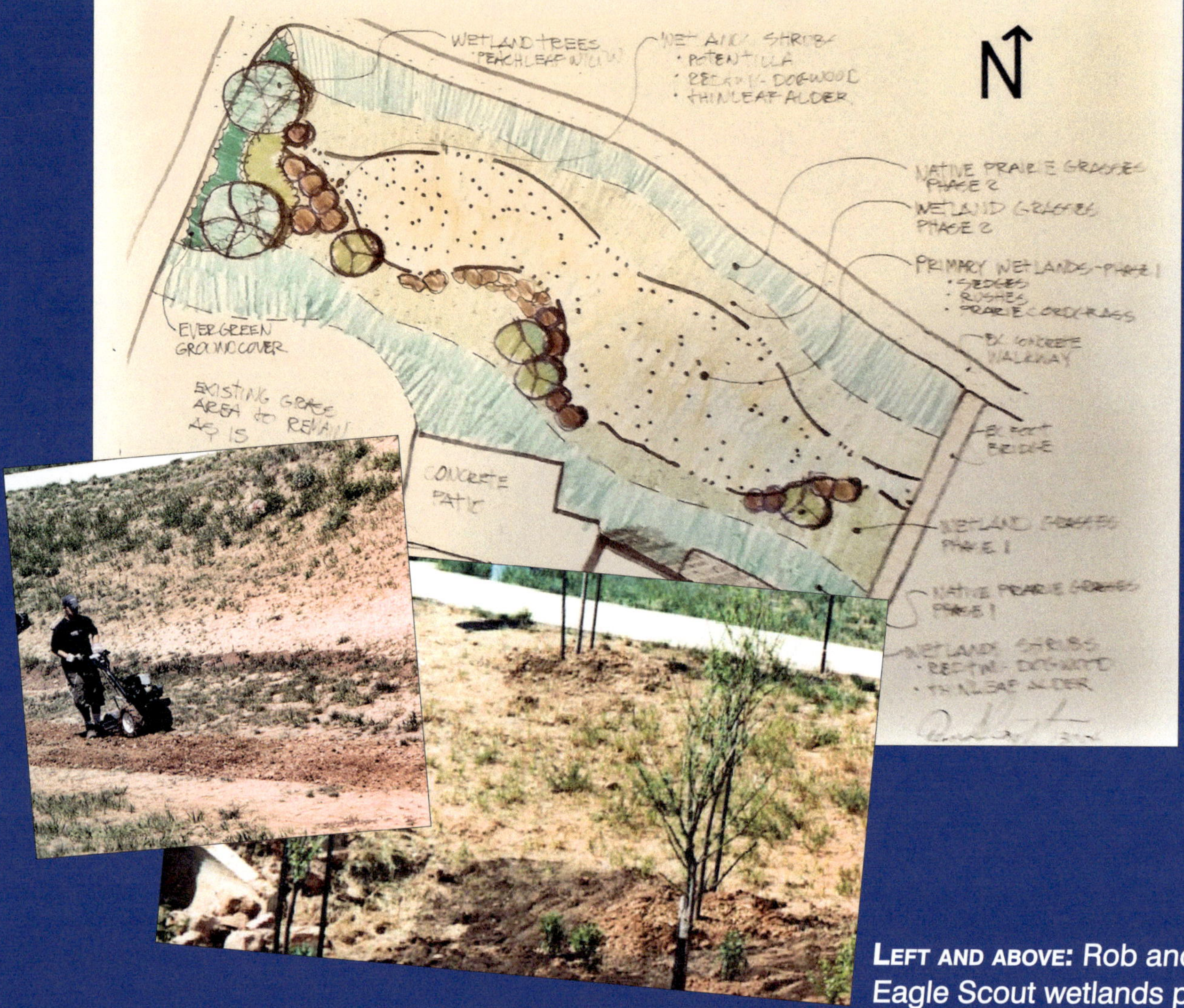

Left and above: Rob and his Eagle Scout wetlands project. **Right:** with the USS Polaris at City Park Lake in Fort Collins. **Right inset:** Rob on finishing welding the USS Polaris.

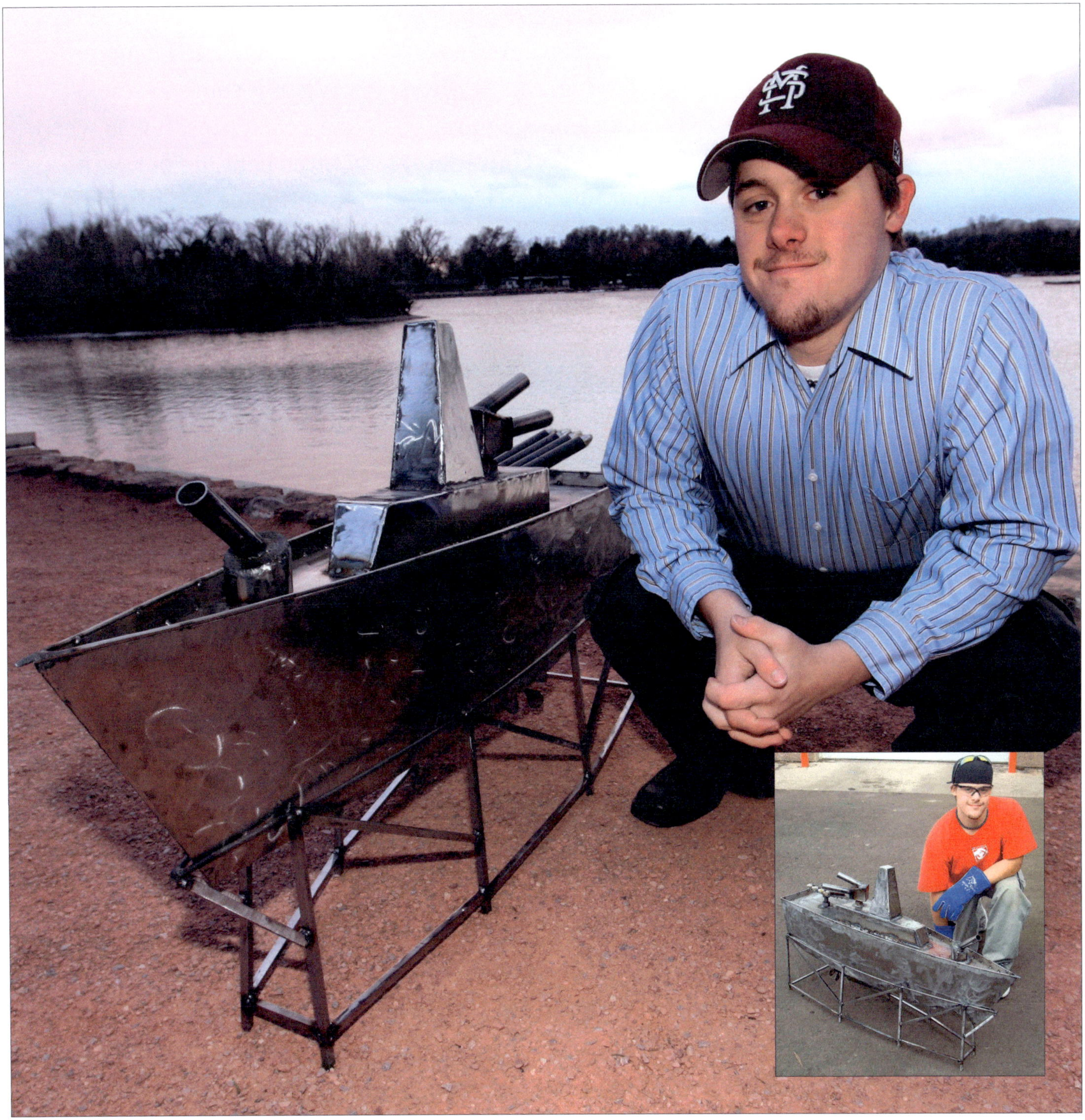

College days

> *Your words and actions today will guide your life tomorrow.*
>
> Rob

I WAS ACCEPTED into the CAD and welding programs at Mesa State College (now Colorado Mesa University) in Grand Junction, Colo., during the fall of my senior year. The 16 credits that I got with the high school welding program counted as 16 college credits.

I started classes at Mesa State in the fall of 2009 and lived in a new dorm. I bussed across town to go to the welding and CAD classes and had my core classes at the main campus. I developed strong friendships with my pod-mates and some of my classmates. I should note that Colorado Voc Rehab helped pay some of my tuition at Mesa State because of my mDs.

During my second year of college in 2010, I decided to try things that were not healthy for my body. The first time I tried tobacco chew, I spit it into a sink, and never tried it again. When it came to smoking cigarettes, it was when I was hanging out with my friends and drinking. I admit smoking was a bad idea, but I tried it several times before I finally decided to call it quits. Overall, I learned the hard lesson that I need to choose my actions wisely. I still drink, but try to do so responsibly.

The other experience that I learned was living by myself. I realized at college that I had to be responsible for my own actions, such as keeping a clean room and managing my own laundry. I learned all those skills growing up, but it was different living on my own. I also learned how to control my spending habits.

It was in May 2011 that I decided to transfer back to the welding program at Front Range Community

College in Fort Collins due to my struggles in college-level math and English. Welding required less of both subjects. I ended up attending FRCC for two years to achieve six welding certificates. I graduated with these in May of 2013. With these certificates and the help of Voc Rehab and my SWAP counselor, I applied and was hired at Distinctive Welding Inc. of Fort Collins in August 2013. I am still employed there, having completed four years in August 2017.

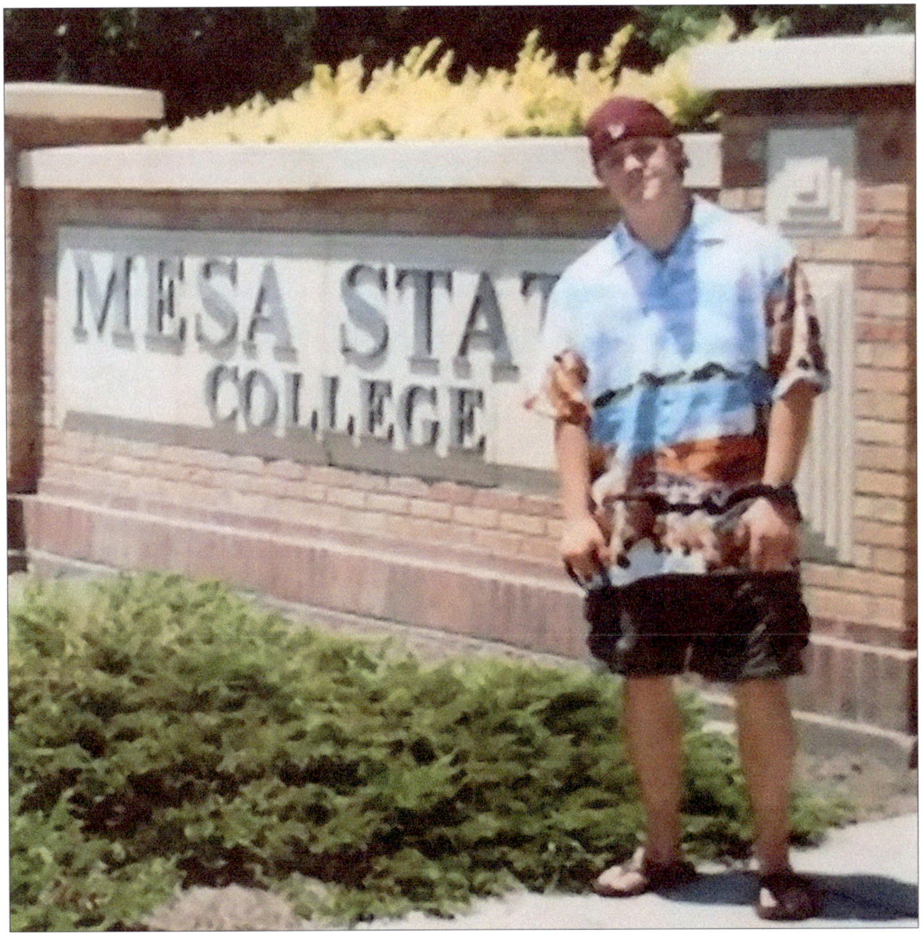

Rob arrives at Mesa State in August 2009.

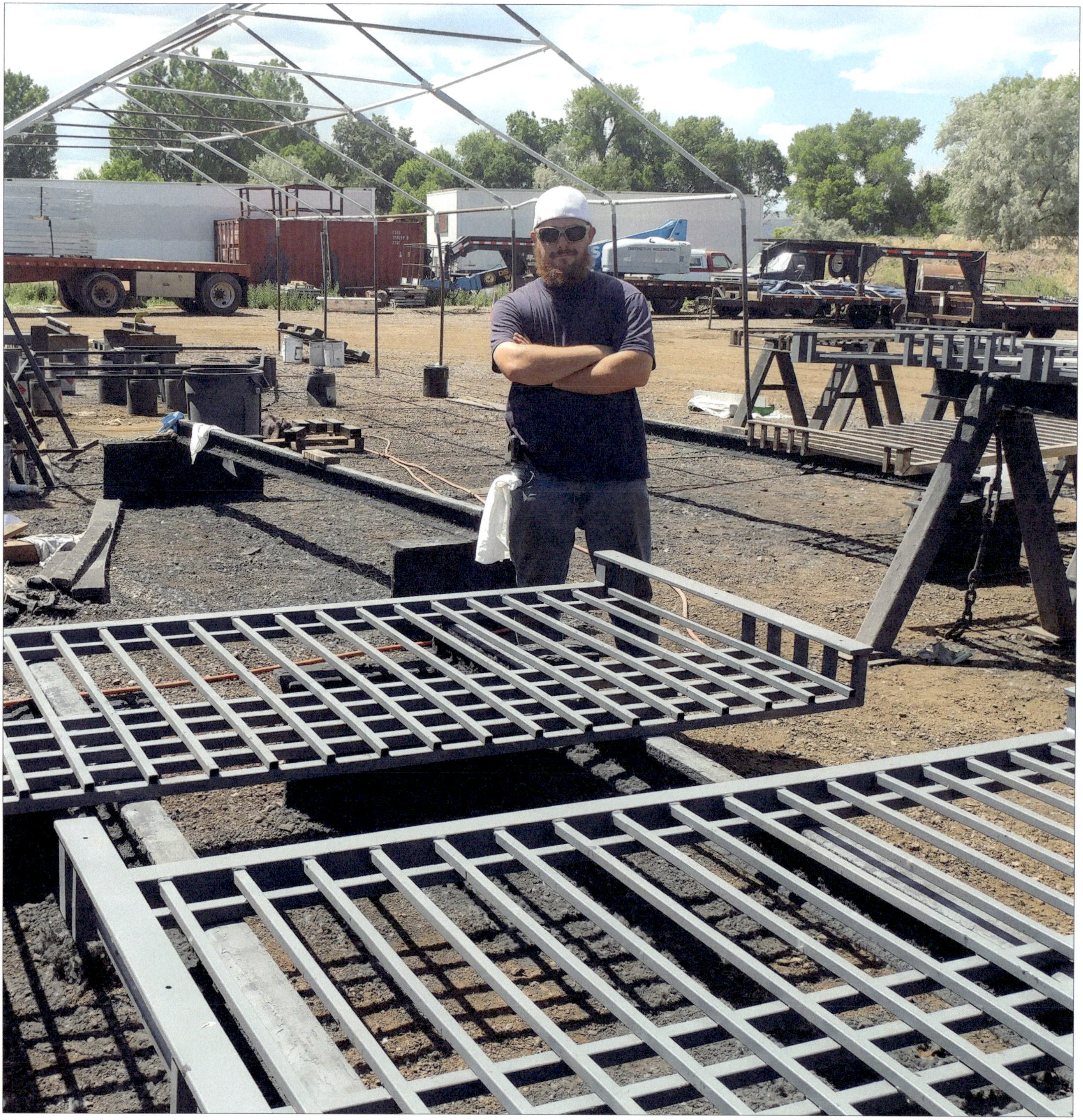

Working in the marketplace

In construction, one learns never to assume that conditions are safe. Check, check, check.
Rob

Rob at the welding yard where he works in Fort Collins.

I STARTED WORKING at Distinctive Welding Inc. in August 2013 as a shop assistant/welder. After awhile I was assigned the task of keeping track of all of the welding consumables.

Welding consumables are welding wire, welding rod, cut-off wheels, 36-grit sanding discs, safety glasses and the like. During my first year, I learned the importance of focusing on my job and not getting distracted. I learned to avoid making excuses as well. I give a lot of credit to my bosses being Christians. **Cory McCormick, Jeremy Hanson** and owner **Caleb Owlsley** have helped me realize the importance of switching from one task to another as the company's priorities dictate.

I have learned how to wipe material down with xylene, which is a strong degreaser designed for metal. Then I would paint it with a structural primer using a paint gun. When I first started doing this, I would experience severe migraines where I was unable to get the job done. Now I seldom have headaches at work. I also do some welding and help with some installations. I have gotten to drive the big trucks to make deliveries and pick up supplies, and drive the forklift in the yard. I have learned the importance of perseverance and determination to get a lot done during a single workday.

I feel like I have learned a lot on my job.

Ministry/ volunteering

> *We... "will give our attention to prayer and the ministry of the word."*
> Acts 6:4 (NIV)

When my brother and I were little and living in Texas, our father led "clipboard" devotionals for us every night so we could discuss life and God.

We each had a clipboard, paper and pencils. We drew pictures to illustrate lessons about life that we pulled from the Bible. We had good discussions.

One night when I was 4, I invited Christ into my heart. This is when I became a Christian. I was 6 when **Pastor Dave Smith** of Northwest Community Church in San Antonio baptized me in a lake.

I also attended a church program called AWANA. It was a ministry designed to equip children with the message of the gospel. I learned how to memorize scriptures and do different games and songs.

Through the years I have been involved in a few different churches and youth programs. After we moved to Fort Collins, my family attended Timberline Church. Casey and I were involved in kids and youth groups.

We both joined the church JOY Team, youth entrusted to teach and train younger kids. There were 40 jobs. I handled the set-up and tear down, some small groups, the activities at the beginning, and the sound and media booth. I came back during college breaks and after college to help out as an adult leader. I plugged in where needed. My biggest job was setting up the stage Saturday afternoon before that night's kids service and the three services on Sunday. After the last service, I tore down the sets and put things away with a team.

I have recently joined Mill City Church in Fort

Collins where my brother Casey is on staff. I help set up and tear down the auditorium each weekend. I also run the camera, computer or lights, depending on where I am needed.

I belong to one of my father's weekly small groups. It's for 20-somethings who share a meal and study the Bible.

Monthly, the group joins a bike team to serve free breakfast to men and women without homes of their own and fix their bikes without charge.

Starting in 2011, I became a self-advocate for individuals with mosaic Down syndrome and Down syndrome, speaking at international conferences.

Over the years, Casey and I participated in numerous mission trips, starting as Teen Missions "Peanuts" in Florida when we were 7 and 9. Later one or both of us served in such places as Belgium, Haiti, Mexico, Guatemala and Hong Kong.

Some of the teams worked construction. We laid rebar, put a roof on a small house, and cleaned bricks so that they could be re-purposed.

On other trips, we showed the JESUS film, ran sports camps, and organized vacation bible schools.

We learned first-hand that the gospel is cross-cultural and to pray for the world.

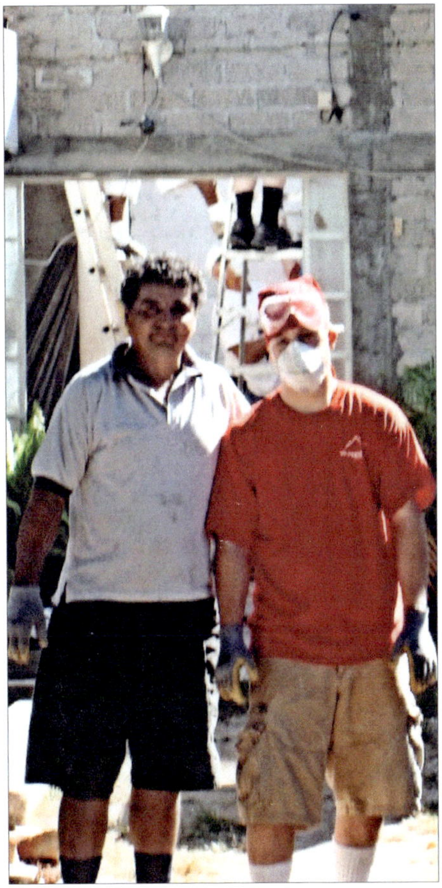

Rob with Pastor Luis on a construction project in Puerto Vallarta, Mexico.

Trials/tests/ triumphs

Consider it pure joy,
my brothers and sisters,
whenever you face trials
of many kinds, because
you know that the testing
of your faith produces
perseverance. Let
perseverance finish its
work so that you may be
mature and complete, not
lacking anything.
James 1:2-4 (NIV)

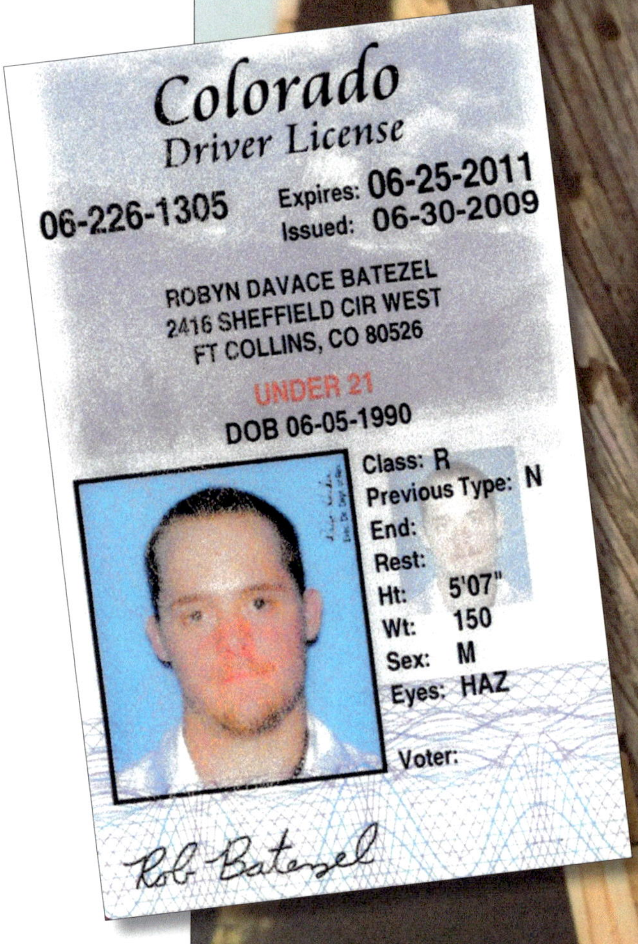

Colorado
Driver License
06-226-1305
Expires: 06-25-2011
Issued: 06-30-2009
ROBYN DAVACE BATEZEL
2416 SHEFFIELD CIR WEST
FT COLLINS, CO 80526
UNDER 21
DOB 06-05-1990
Class: R
Previous Type: N
End:
Rest:
Ht: 5'07"
Wt: 150
Sex: M
Eyes: HAZ
Voter:
Rob Batezel

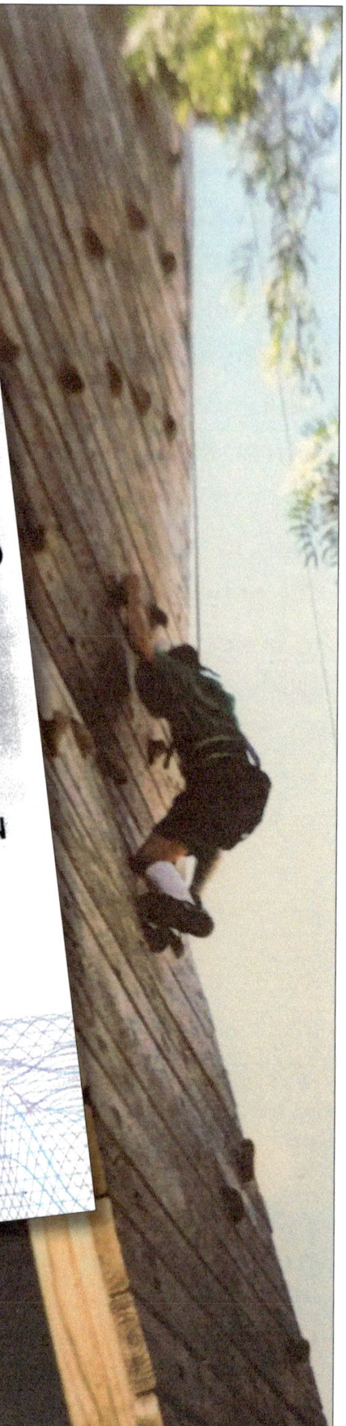

Far left: Rob's hard-earned drivers license.
Left: Rob ascending a climbing wall at a church retreat in Texas.

Growing up with mDs, I knew some things would be easy for me and others things harder.

I earned the rank of Eagle Scout right before my 16th birthday. At 18, I graduated from high school even though, when I was little, few people thought high school graduation was a realistic goal.

But there were discouragements as well. I had to accept that I wasn't cut out for military service due to my mDs. This was disappointing because many members of my family had served in the military, some for full careers.

Overall, perseverance paid off. An example is the time it took to earn my drivers license. I started with an intense drivers education program that specialized in defensive driving. But I was told it would take me hundreds of training hours to get a license due to mDs.

Fortunately, folks at the **Center for Neurorehabilitation** in Fort Collins said they could help. First, I had to pass a written test to get a learner's permit. I could take the test only five times per year. I studied hard and passed the written test on the fifth time!

Then the neurorehab folks gave me several months of occupational therapy to improve my binocularity and response time. I took regular drivers education and prepared for the actual driving test. The limit was five tests over a lifetime. Thankfully, I passed the test on the third try!

I waited until I was 19 to take the driving test because I didn't feel confident to drive by myself before then. This was a huge step of independence for me. At first I drove our family cars, but eventually I bought a used SUV.

My parents were open about my mDs diagnosis early on, but I didn't advertise it until sixth grade when I did a health fair project on mDs. This was when I first heard about the International Mosaic Down Syndrome Association (imdsa.org). I went to my first conference after graduating from high school. Since then, I have been to conferences in Orlando, Fla., San Antonio, Williamsburg, Va., and Boston. I am a self-advocate for the organization and speak at the conferences.

I'm also involved in my local Northern Colorado Down Syndrome Association.

Gratitude

> *"It is your family that will get you through the struggles of life."*
>
> Rob

I AM GRATEFUL for a huge family of supporters. My parents ushered me into faith in Christ. Mom helped me with speech and language, and Dad coached me with English literacy. Both challenged me to earn the rank of Eagle Scout and spurred me on to educational goals and a good job.

My younger brother and best friend **Casey** has always had my back. Early on, he was always able to explain things in ways I could understand. As adults, I'm thankful we can work together on his home renovations and church projects.

I also credit my **Aunt Suzie** and **Uncle John** for "telling it to me straight." Uncle John, who can fix anything, has always given me good advice. He taught me how to change the oil in my car. Aunt Suzie helped me realize that I am in control of my destiny.

I also relish time I spend with my extended family. My cousin **Amber** and her husband **Tyler** live nearby with their four children, **Trinity, Mick, Dierdre** and **Kellen.** My cousin **Kevin,** a lawyer, recently moved nearby. I don't get to see my other relatives much except at reunions.

Every step along the way, God has provided the right people at the right time. Doctors, teachers, Scout leaders, pastors and friends encouraged me to plug away.

My deepest thanks to all (you know who you are)! I wouldn't be where I am today without you!

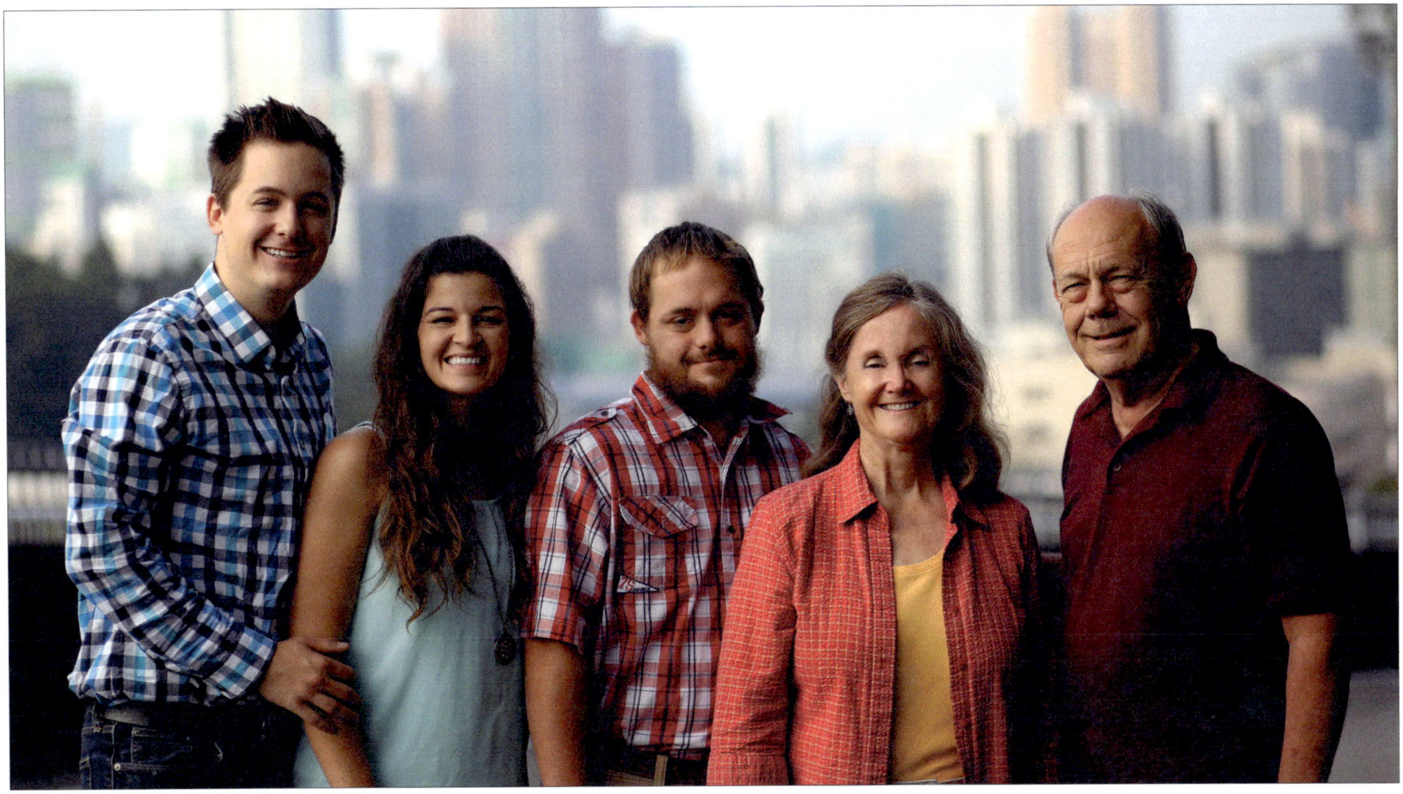

Epilogue

> *"I hope and pray that this book can be an example of how to be a light in today's society."*
> Rob

The Batezel family in Hong Kong in fall 2016. From left, Casey and his wife, Lindsay, Rob, Roxanne and Tony.

"Blessed are the peacemakers, for they will be called children of God."

Matthew 5:9 (NIV)

"You are the light of the world. A town built on a hill cannot be hidden. Neither do people light a lamp and put it under a bowl. Instead they put it on its stand, and it gives light to everyone in the house. In the same way, let your light shine before others, that they may see your good deeds and glorify your Father in heaven.

Matthew 5:14-16 (NIV)